How To Become A Successful Healthcare Entrepreneur

How To Become A Successful Healthcare Entrepreneur

FOR DOCTORS AND HEALTHCARE PROFESSIONALS IN NIGERIA

● ● ●

Dr. J. Adeghe MBBS, PhD, FRCOG.

ISBN-13: 9781533328861
ISBN-10: 1533328862

Table of Contents

About the Author

● ● ●

DR. JUDE-HARRIS ADEGHE, MBBS, PhD, FRCOG, is a consultant in obstetrics, gynecology, and reproductive medicine and a successful healthcare entrepreneur. He is the CEO of St. Jude Hospitals and Clinics, which has hospitals in the United Kingdom and Nigeria.

Dr. Adeghe graduated from the University of Nigeria Medical School, Enugu, Nigeria. Following graduation, he came to the United Kingdom to pursue specialist training in obstetrics and gynecology and research in assisted reproductive technology, which led to the award of a PhD by the University of Birmingham, United Kingdom. He also obtained Membership of the Royal College of Obstetricians and Gynaecologists (MRCOG).

He rose to the top of his career as a National Health Service (NHS) consultant over a period of ten years before leaving the NHS to set up his own hospital, St. Jude's Women's Hospital in Wolverhampton, United Kingdom, a bold entrepreneurial move. He is well established as a skilled clinician and successful healthcare entrepreneur.

Dr. Adeghe is married and blessed with three children.

Introduction

● ● ●

Unlock new solutions to local challenges.

—Barack Obama, *On his visit to Kenya in July 2015*

A legendary hero is usually the founder of something—the founder
of a new age, the founder of a new religion, the founder of a new
city, the founder of a new way of life. In order to found something
new, one has to leave the old and go on a quest of the seed idea, a
germinal idea that has the potential of bringing forth that new thing.

—Joseph Campbell, *Hero with a Thousand Faces*

The above is, in my view, the true entrepreneurial creed.

The idea of writing a book on healthcare entrepreneurship first occurred to me about four years ago, but the practicality of running my healthcare businesses relegated the idea to the background. My frequent visits to Nigeria in the last couple of years have rekindled my desire to write this book for several reasons:

1. I believe that entrepreneurial creativity in healthcare can contribute immensely to improving the sorry state of health services in Nigeria.

2. While entrepreneurial healthcare setups are relatively commonplace in Nigeria, they all seem to maintain the status quo, rather than being creative and unique.

3. Healthcare-service provision in the majority of other African countries is mainly left almost entirely to the government to develop, and consistently, the various governments in Africa have made a right mess of it.

I believe that entrepreneurial activities in the healthcare arena have a vital role to play in expanding the scope and improving the quality of healthcare services. Privately owned healthcare facilities are many and varied in Nigeria and in many other African countries. Many of these facilities—medical clinics, medical laboratory services, physiotherapy clinics, and pharmacies—are virtually carbon copies of each other. This is not necessarily a bad thing, but the Nigerian healthcare arena is crying out for innovation and creativity that will positively impact service delivery and health outcomes. Most medical clinics operate as jacks-of-all-trades, offering services in all specialties. There is no culture of referring cases that fall outside of their training and skills to another doctor who is better placed to help in that case. There seems to be a herd mentality among healthcare professionals, most of them focusing in the perceived lucrative specialties—gynecology, maternity, surgery, fertility, and in vitro fertilization. There are very few private clinics focusing mainly on primary healthcare, and yet this is one area that will impact positively on the health of the population. According to Bill Gates, access to primary care is the foundation of good health.

Teaching and encouraging entrepreneurship is not part of the standard curriculum in the medical sciences. As far as I can ascertain, there are no guidebooks about how to establish a private healthcare facility or that stress the importance of innovation and creativity in health-service provision.

As already stated, I have three reasons for writing this book:

1. To highlight the important role of entrepreneurship in healthcare improvement in both the scope and the quality of service delivery

2. To provide a guide for healthcare professionals who wish to set up a private practice
3. To stress the need for every practice to be creative and innovative in the types of services provided and how the service is delivered

When most people think of healthcare, the first thing that probably springs to mind is a doctor's clinic. However, healthcare service goes well beyond that. I wrote this book for doctors and other healthcare professionals including dentists, nurses, medical-laboratory scientists, pharmacists, physiotherapists, radiologists, optometrists, opticians, and others. This book outlines basic principles that apply to all specialties.

Some may see the title of this book and ask, "Why focus on Africa? Surely entrepreneurial skills and principles are the same the world over." If you are thinking this, you are correct, but, as they say, it is "horses for courses." Healthcare priorities are different in Africa than in the Western world. The healthcare challenges prevalent in Nigeria and other countries in Africa need solutions that require an understanding of local cultural and socioeconomic factors. Many of these challenges are nonexistent in the Western world. The socioeconomic factors and the infrastructure problems prevalent in Africa deserve special mention and attention, and they require innovative and creative entrepreneurial skills.

CHAPTER 1

What Is Healthcare Entrepreneurship?

● ● ●

Entrepreneurs are ordinary people with extraordinary determination.

—Philip and Sandra Webb

The starting point of all achievements is desire.

—Napoleon Hill

An entrepreneur is an innovator, a job creator, a
game-changer, a business leader, a disruptor, an adventurer.

—Richard Branson

What Is a Healthcarepreneur?

Healthcarepreneur is a term I coined to describe a healthcare practitioner who is entrepreneurial within his or her specialist area or any entrepreneur whose activity is within the healthcare arena. So a healthcarepreneur is basically an entrepreneur. A doctor entrepreneur may be referred to as a *doctorpreneur.*

The English word "entrepreneur" is derived from the French word *entreprendre,* which means "to undertake." Another meaning is "business manager." The term dates from between 1875 and 1880.

Definitions of an entrepreneur include the following:

- A person who organizes a business venture and assumes the risk for it
- An employer of productive labor
- The owner or manager of a business enterprise who, by risk and initiative, attempts to make profits
- A middleman or commercial intermediary

Luke Johnson, a notable English entrepreneur, in an article titled *"Don't run a business if you can't even run your own life"* (The Sunday Times, Business Section, England, 7th June 2015) listed the following traits of an entrepreneur :

- Ambition
- Appetite for risk
- Industry
- Persistence
- Numeracy
- Creativity
- Self-confidence
- Optimism
- Grit
- Self-discipline

Luke Johnson asserts that if there is one defining attribute above all others that makes for a successful entrepreneur, it is self-discipline. He says, "Possess this and all other qualities are secondary." I could not agree more.

Note that "intrapreneur" means something very different. An intrapreneur is an employee of a large corporation who is given the freedom and financial support to create new products, services, or systems and does not have to follow the corporation's usual routines and protocols.

What is Healthcare?

Your health is your greatest wealth

Healthcare is defined as "the diagnosis, treatment, and prevention of disease, illness, injury, and other physical and mental impairments in human beings."

Healthcare has many branches. It includes medicine, dentistry, nursing, midwifery, pharmacy, laboratory science, psychology, optometry, and many more. Within each specialty are several subspecialist areas. For example, within the surgical specialty are general surgery, orthopedics, neurosurgery, heart surgery, and others. Obstetrics and gynecology have myriad subspecialist areas. It is evident, therefore, that healthcare constitutes a wide area of different skills.

Healthcare delivery depends on highly trained practitioners, and services are provided through a system that is often layered into primary care, secondary care, and tertiary care. However, these demarcations often are not clearly distinct. Public health is frequently regarded as another layer, but it actually blends across primary, secondary, and tertiary levels. This is because public health is concerned mainly with the entire population and focuses on disease prevention, health promotion, and prolongation of life across all groups.

Healthcare Challenges in Africa

What often highlights the huge healthcare problems in Africa and brings it to the fore is when there is an epidemic so severe that it causes international concern. For example, the 2014 Ebola outbreak extended beyond Africa but was contained to one or two cases in the United States and the United Kingdom. The ease with which epidemics spread in Africa and the developing world is underpinned by widespread poverty, poor socioeconomic conditions, poor water supplies, poor housing, few and inadequately equipped hospitals, high levels of illiteracy, and inadequate healthcare funding.

The healthcare challenges in Africa have been researched and commented upon exhaustively and are the subject of many books and theses. The main factors thought to contribute to poor healthcare provision in Nigeria and other African countries are as follows: (1) inadequate funding of healthcare, (2) corruption, (3) inadequate staffing, (4) no effective regulation of healthcare providers, (5) poor physical infrastructure, (6) lack of power supply, (7) poor water supply, and (8) counterfeit drugs.

The consequences of the problems listed above include the following:

- Unacceptably high infant and maternal mortality rates: According to UNICEF data published in 2013, Nigeria has the second-highest child (under five) and maternal mortality rates in the world. According to these figures, a woman's chance of dying from pregnancy and childbirth in Nigeria is 1 in 13. In the UK, the figure is 1 in 10,000. The infant mortality rate in Nigeria (2014 data) is 71.50 per 1000 live births; the corresponding UK figure is 3.8 deaths per 1000 live births (2013).
- Frequent epidemics of infectious diseases: recent cases in point include Ebola and Lassa fever.
- Healthcare brain drain: This is a term used to describe the emigration of Nigerian doctors and other healthcare professionals to the United Kingdom, Europe, the United States, and Saudi Arabia to seek better career prospects and financial gains.

As the twentieth-century Yorkshire expression says, "Where there is muck, there is brass," meaning that where there are dirty jobs to be done, there is money to be made. This rings true in the healthcare situation in Nigeria and Africa. The numerous problems provide a fertile ground for entrepreneurial innovation and creativity.

The World Health Organization (WHO) recommends that 11 percent of a country's budget should be allocated to the healthcare sector. In Nigeria, only 3.8 percent was allocated to healthcare in 2013, which represents serious underfunding. There are also issues with how the healthcare allocation is managed, given the endemic corruption in the country. Typically, a large portion of healthcare funds is embezzled. Compared to many African countries, Nigeria with her oil resources can be considered a rich nation. Therefore, inadequate healthcare funding is entirely unacceptable.

CHAPTER 2

Self-Evaluation: Creative Career Planning

● ● ●

Few joys are comparable to that of launching
and building your business.

—Laurie Beth Jones

Vision without action is a daydream; action
without vision is a nightmare.

—Japanese Proverb

Paid Employment or Entrepreneurial Self-Employment?

This is the question that many healthcare professionals have to consider at some point. You may be reading this and saying to yourself, "I don't have to choose. I'll do both." This is a valid comment, and this is indeed what many doctors and other healthcare professionals do. The typical hospital consultant in Nigeria holds a post in a teaching hospital or general hospital and also has a private clinic outside of the hospital where he or she practices in the evenings after normal working hours. On the face of it, this model seems to work well and appears to be the equivalent of getting the best of both worlds. However, this model raises several concerns including conflict of interest, possible breach of employment contract, and divided attention, all of which may impact quality of care in both settings.

Paid employment in a government hospital provides a high degree of job security and peace of mind. In most cases, the healthcare professional has a job for life with a defined career progression pathway. As long as the doctor performs well and does nothing egregious to lose the job, he or she can generally be sure of a monthly salary. However, payment of salaries is not necessarily a given in Nigeria. Nonpayment of salaries is a common reason for Nigerian healthcare professionals going on strike. In paid employment, apart from the practitioner's professional duties and accountability, the buck stops with the owners of the hospital, typically the government or other organization. The practitioner does not have to be concerned with the hiring or firing of staff or the risks inherent in running a business. On the other hand, you do not have full control of your destiny, and the potential for financial progression is limited. You know the top of your salary scale at the top of your career ladder. It has been said that "a job will never make you rich," although one could add the proviso, "unless you are making shrewd investments with your salary." If you are a creative person, a salaried job alone may not give you a platform to express your creativity to the fullest.

In contrast to paid employment, entrepreneurial self-employment involves the risk and uncertainty inherent in a new business. It also requires unrelenting hard work. However, it gives you a platform to control your destiny and to express your creativity and skills. In addition, you are able to reap the rich rewards that may follow. You have the opportunity to achieve personal fulfillment by impacting the lives of your service users in a positive way. Moreover, you will create jobs for many people, and finally, you will leave your footsteps in the sands of time in your professional arena. In the words of Philip and Sandra Webb, "The feeling of self-worth that you develop as a business owner far outweighs everything else."

Which is better—paid employment or entrepreneurial self-employment? One is not necessarily better than the other. For most people, it is ultimately a question of which option suits their personality type and aspirations.

The first step to becoming an entrepreneur is self-evaluation. This is a process of "career soul searching." You need to review where you are in your career path and carefully and honestly assess your skills and attributes.

NEWLY QUALIFIED PRACTITIONERS

For example, any young Nigerian doctor who has completed his or her internship and national youth service and who is considering entrepreneurship should carry out a detailed self-evaluation. This should include a process of career review and planning and self-assessment for traits suited to entrepreneurship. Relevant questions should include the following:

- Are you ready for entrepreneurship? To meaningfully consider entrepreneurship this early in your career, you should have a unique product or innovative service that you hope to deliver.
- Is your professional experience adequate for your proposed venture?
- Are you better off pursuing specialist training in your chosen field prior to pursuing entrepreneurship?
- Do you have the general traits that will help your entrepreneurial pursuit? These include ambition, appetite for risk, industry, persistence, numeracy, creativity, self-confidence, optimism, and grit.
- In particular, do you have the necessary self-discipline? According to Luke Johnson, if there is one defining attribute above all others that marks a successful entrepreneur, it is self-discipline. Possess this and all other qualities are secondary. He quotes President Harry Truman: "In reading the lives of great men, I found that the first victory they won was over themselves…self-discipline came first." Johnson concludes, "Develop self-discipline and the world is your oyster."

For the newly qualified and certified dentist, pharmacist, nurse, medical laboratory scientist, physiotherapist, optician, or optometrist, the above self-evaluation plan applies as well.

Experienced Practitioners

For those healthcare practitioners who have been qualified for some time and are at career crossroads, the relevant issues may be more specific than those outlined above. For example, the questions relating to limited experience in their fields of practice may not be applicable. In general, they are likely to have sufficient experience to back up their service offerings. However, they need to perform in-depth self-evaluations relating to the personal attributes listed above. Consider these additional questions:

- Do you feel fulfilled in your present job? If not, do you believe you can achieve self-fulfillment through service and self-expression?
- Are you motivated to take risks? Risk is inherent in entrepreneurship.
- Are you resilient in the pursuit of your goals? The road to entrepreneurial success can be tough and lonely.
- Are you adaptable? It is a big change from being part of an established organization to being your own boss.
- Are you ready to take responsibility? As an employee in an establishment, responsibility for the day-to-day running of the business lies with management. When you are your own boss, you are responsible for everything. Entrepreneurs must take full responsibility for making things happen and rectifying any problems that may occur.
- Are you a good leader? Your entrepreneurial journey will require leadership skills in putting a team together and leading it with purpose.
- What motivates you? You must be clear about your motivation for embarking on the entrepreneurial pathway. Your motivation will to a large extent shape the nature and structure of your venture. You may be motivated by one or more of the PERFECT work motivations described by G. Richard Shell in his book *Success, Your Way: Do What You're Meant to Do.*
  - Personal growth and development
  - Entrepreneurial independence
  - Religious or spiritual identity
  - Family

o Expressing yourself through ideas, invention, or the arts
o Community—serving a cause, helping people in need
o Talent-based striving for excellence

The essence of self-evaluation is a sort of creative career-planning process. Career planning is applying your God-given skills in an area or a field that captures your passion, with the sole aim of solving a problem in that area of endeavor. Creative career planning involves being proactive rather than simply being active. When the principles of creative career planning have been embraced and applied, you will be ready for an impactful entrepreneurial venture.

According to Shell, "When you are engaged in an activity that feels especially suited to you (i.e., it fits your key personality traits), very little friction is generated between your capabilities and whatever you are doing. You are likely to experience what positive psychologists call 'flow'—a sense of absorption in your activity that causes you to lose track of time and perform whatever you are doing at your highest level of skill."

Perhaps the vital points of self-evaluation can best be captured in Napoleon Hill's Personal Success Equation, which is as follows:

Your Personal Success = {(P + T) x A x Ac} + F
P = Passion; T = Talent; A = Right Association; Ac = Right Action;
F = Faith in Yourself and Your Mission

To conclude this chapter, I want to quote Brad Feld, author of *Feldthought— Burning Entrepreneur*: "When launching or growing a start-up, the first thing to start up is your attitude. You must be on fire, on the edge, and on the attack silently. With this personality mashup, you'll be a burning entrepreneur."

CHAPTER 3

Generating Innovative Ideas

One idea can change your future.

—ROGER SHOHANA

73% of product innovations come from market needs,
whereas 27% come from technological opportunities.

—URBAN AND HAUSER, *DESIGN AND MARKETING OF NEW PRODUCTS*

To live a creative life, we must lose our fear of being wrong.

—JOSEPH CHILTON PEARCE

Creativity has to do with the ability to question.

—MICHAEL RAY AND ROCHELLE MYERS, *CREATIVITY IN BUSINESS*

HOW DO YOU GENERATE A healthcare-business idea? This is at the core of the entrepreneurial process. You may already have an idea or a plan. As you look around at many healthcare businesses, you may find that they all seem to be a "rubber stamp." For example, many hospitals or clinics in Nigeria offer a similar range of services, and those services are delivered in the same way. The doctors who own these hospitals are all typically financially successful and provide valuable services in their communities. However, the poor state of healthcare services in Africa and the developing world suggests that there is a need to do things differently. The situation cries out for innovation, but new entrants to the healthcare entrepreneurial arena risk playing perpetual second fiddle to the older and more established setups.

The following principles, when applied to your business ideas, will help to set your venture apart from others and ensure success:

1. Adopt a problem-centered approach to generating and developing your healthcare business idea. As a healthcare practitioner, you no doubt are already aware of the shortcomings of the services that are already available. If for any reason you are not fully aware, visiting some of the existing hospitals or clinics will enlighten you on the status quo.
2. Question the status quo. Can it be done better?
3. List what you see as the most significant shortcomings or problems in the hospitals or clinics as they are today. Which single item on your list do you think will make the best or biggest impact in your community and beyond?
4. To have a competitive advantage, any healthcare start-up must have a "unique selling point," or a USP. The USP may be involve any of the following:
   • Service type
   • Mode of service delivery
   • Cost of service
   • Point of service delivery

PRACTICAL STEPS TO TAKE
   • Think, and think again. Think outside of the box.
   • Write down your ideas. Remember that your ideas should be based on a better way of doing things. Don't just write, "I want to start a

clinic." That is not good enough. Remember that you need to set yourself apart from the crowd.

- Next, write down how your idea will make a difference to users of the service you propose to set up. This may mean doing an established service better or providing a service that is not widely available but is very much needed in your community.
- If your idea is based on a new "product" or a new way to deliver service, has it been validated by an independent body or other credible practitioners?
- Discuss your ideas with confidants. Your confidants may be trusted colleagues, friends, or family. Note their comments carefully, including any possible criticisms.
- Think things over for a period of time—days, weeks, or for as long as you need in order to be certain that your ideas will remain exciting to you.

At this point, you need to develop a business plan.

CHAPTER 4

Plan and Strategize

● ● ●

When you fail to plan, you plan to fail.

—Benjamin Franklin

Write the vision; make it plain upon tables,
that he may run that readeth it.

—Habakkuk 2:2

Planning is like a map. If you take the time to plan your route
before you set off, you can save a lot of time along the way.

—Philip and Sandra Webb

Having developed your idea for a healthcare entrepreneurial start-up, the next step is to write a business plan for the actualization of your idea. Developing and implementing your idea are the keys to success. Writing your plan is not a one-day exercise. It should take place over a period of time, and there is no hard-and-fast rule on how long it should take. The important thing is that it should be meticulous. Remember, it is your road map.

The average healthcare practitioner, whether newly qualified or established in a job, is unlikely to have any experience in business-plan writing. It is a good idea to use business-planning software to help you produce a plan for your healthcare start-up. Also, reading the business plans written by other people may be helpful. You can review some examples at www.bplans.co.uk, a website that focuses on medical and healthcare business plans. One good business-plan application that I strongly recommend is Business Plan Pro. You can find out more about this software at www.paloalto.com/uk.

It is not the purpose of this chapter to delve into the details of business-plan writing, but I will highlight what I consider to be the core elements of an effective healthcare business plan. Suffice it to say that it should be inspirational, structured, well thought out, and based on your vision and your plans and procedures to build your healthcare business. It defines what you want to achieve and how.

The content of a good business plan should include the following elements.

Your Title Page

This will include the name of your proposed healthcare business.

Your Mission or Vision Statement

Simply put, your mission or vision statement is the declaration of your healthcare business intent. It should be carefully, meaningfully, and crisply crafted, and it must encapsulate the raison d'être of your business. As described by Philip and Sandra Webb, your mission or vision statement "is a motivational statement as well as a descriptive statement and contains some of the emotion that will bind the business together as it moves forward."

For example, the mission statement of my fertility clinic is "Effective Fertility Care Delivered with Compassion and Honesty." I felt that effectiveness is key when conducting investigations and performing treatments for couples experiencing difficulty conceiving. Infertility is well known to generate stress and anxiety in affected couples. Therefore, showing compassion and honesty are key features of our service.

Another example is the mission statement of Smith and Nephew, a global medical technology company specializing in surgical devices for orthopedics and devices for wound management. Their mission statement is "To Help Improve People's Lives." This is a realistic, yet broad, objective to describe what they do.

An Overview of Your Business

This section should provide a description of your profession or specialty, discussing the services you will offer. You should also say a few words about the importance of your services, obvious as it might be.

Your Background

This is a very important section. It highlights your educational and career background, your special skills, and why you are best equipped to make a success of your start-up. It should be a brief CV outlining the jobs and positions you have held throughout your career.

Services You Provide and Your Unique Selling Points

Describe your service or product, emphasizing its value or purpose. Emphasize what makes your service or product different from others. In so doing, you are defining your unique selling points (USPs). In what specific ways will the user of your service or product benefit?

Goals

Define your short-term goals, what you want to achieve over the next two to four years. These objectives should be clear and conform to the SMART criteria for setting goals. SMART stands for specific, measurable, achievable, realistic, and timely. These objectives will form the benchmarks against which you can measure your progress going forward.

SERVICES AND COSTS

You should include a list of services you plan to offer together with the price for each service. It is important to establish prices early rather than deciding as you go along. The price list should be included in your service users' guide to help ensure a professional image for your business. Be sure, however, that your prices are both realistic and competitive.

CASH-FLOW PROJECTION

This is important for sound financial planning. It will illustrate how your overhead costs will be covered and identify any need for borrowing from a bank or an investor. If you need to borrow from a bank, they will need to see a good business plan with good cash-flow projections. You may need help from an accountant to write your cash-flow projections.

SWOT ANALYSIS

It is a good idea to include an analysis of the strengths, weaknesses, opportunities, and threats (SWOT) regarding your business. This is useful for both the initial planning and ongoing development of your business.

The business plan should not be merely a paper exercise to discard once your business is up and running. You should revisit it regularly to see how you are progressing toward your goals.

PREMISES, EQUIPMENT, AND UTILITIES

Securing suitable premises is very important for the success of your start-up healthcare business. While a purpose-built facility is ideal, that is probably not a realistic goal for most start-ups. The ideal facility is one that is accessible and offers appropriate floor space for your type of healthcare business. Internal restructuring and refurbishment of an existing building may be required. You must give careful consideration to your specific requirements. In addition, close attention should be paid to the décor and the cleanliness of the interior and exterior of the facility. First impressions matter. The premises must be secure, ideally with a perimeter wall or fencing to provide clear demarcation from surrounding buildings as well as a first line of security. This will also provide your clients a sense of privacy and confidentiality.

Purchasing up-to-date equipment is a key factor in delivering a first-class service. You may need to negotiate a bank loan to help purchase everything that you require in this regard. This is where a good business plan will be helpful, as your lender will want to see it.

It is common knowledge in Nigeria that the electricity supply is unreliable. Therefore, one essential requirement is a generator. The generator is supposed to provide backup, but depending on the nature of your service—for example if you provide electricity-critical medical services—you may find that you are using the generator more than the normal electricity supply. The situation with the water supply is just as bad. You will certainly need a borehole, as do most households and businesses.

STAFFING

Ultimately, the quality of your service delivery will be only as good as your staff. Therefore, be sure to take time to seek out well-qualified staff for different roles in the business. You will have to pay more, but it will be well worth it. Poor staffing will constitute a drag on the progress of your business. Competition in the business world is very tough, and only high-quality service delivered by well-trained staff will set you apart from others. Think twice before employing your brother, cousin, or any relative just because they are your relatives. As P. J. Daniels says, "It may be better for you and your business if you give such relatives some pocket money to stay at home."

Apart from the core healthcare professionals that will be working with you, you will need others to give your business a sound footing. These include a receptionist, an administrative staff person, a cleaner, and a security officer. There must be a clear job description for each member of the staff and clear definition of roles. At the start-up stage, it may not be financially feasible to appoint more than one or two support staff. In this case, those you do hire should be prepared to multitask. You should also identify an accountant to advise you on bookkeeping and to prepare your accounts and tax returns. Such arrangements are typically on a fee-for-service basis.

REGULATORY REQUIREMENTS

Be sure to register your business with the Corporate Affairs Commission (CAC) and Federal Inland Revenue Service (FIRS). For more information, you should visit their websites, www.new.cac.gov.ng and www.firs.gov.ng, respectively.

It is essential that you follow all relevant requirements for registration and regulation.

CHAPTER 5

Organizational Structure and Governance

● ● ●

Entrepreneur is one who operates, organizes, or
assumes the risks for a business venture

—Anonymous

In the end, we are the sum-total of our actions. Day by day we
write our destiny; for inexorably we become what we do.

—Madame Chiang Kai-Shek

For any entrepreneurial start-up to succeed and flourish, there must be clear systems in place. This is what will create order, efficiency, and quality in your business, and ultimately, this is what will drive profitability. What has been described so far can be likened to the "hardware" of your business. Without the software or operating system, however, the hardware cannot function, or certainly not in a productive way. The software of your business is its organizational structure and governance. An *organizational structure* defines how your business activities, such as job roles, coordination, and supervision, are carried out toward the achievement of business goals. *Organizational governance* is the set of processes, protocols, and policies that determine how the business is run.

A well-planned and well-executed operational structure and governance will lead to quality output. You must make sure that your business adheres to all the rules of the organization. Therefore, continuous monitoring is essential in order to ensure proper implementation. A well-organized business commands the respect of your service users and other stakeholders. Over time, you will earn a reputation for excellence, which will make you more likely to gain patronage locally and internationally.

Important components discussed in this section include the following:

- Statement of purpose and mission statement
- Clients' guide
- Clinical governance
- SoPs (standard operating procedures) for *all* your services and processes
- Quality-management system and a quality manual

Statement of Purpose

This is a description of what you do, where you do it, and whom you do it for. It should include your mission statement, your aims and objectives, the services you provide, how your service meets the needs of your clients, your contact details, the location of your service, and the legal entity of your business.

Clients' Guide

This should contain your statement of purpose and other important information about your business to help inform those who use your services. Such information should include a list of all staff and their roles, your unique selling points, your open hours, and your complaints procedures. The clients' guide can serve as promotional material for your business. Every client or potential client should be given a copy.

CLINICAL GOVERNANCE

Your healthcare business must have at its core a clinical-governance framework. *Clinical governance* is a systematic approach to maintaining and improving the quality of patient care within a health system. It was originally brought into practice within the UK National Health Service (NHS) in 1995 when an anesthetist exposed a high mortality rate for pediatric cardiac surgery at the Bristol Royal Infirmary.

The main pillars of clinical governance are as follows:

- Risk management
- Clinical audit
- Education, training, and continuous professional development
- Evidence-based care and effectiveness
- Clients' experiences and involvement
- Staffing and staff development

It is not the remit of this book to delve into them in detail. Recommended books, websites, and sources of further information are listed under Suggested Reading.

STANDARD OPERATING PROCEDURE (SoP)

SoP is a step-by-step guide for routine procedures carried out in the business. It helps to achieve consistency of performance, efficiency, and quality output.

QUALITY MANAGEMENT SYSTEM (QMS)

This is a document consisting of policies, processes, and procedures to help the business achieve set quality objectives, mainly to consistently meet your clients' expectations and minimize risk.

CHAPTER 6

Quality Assurance in Your Healthcare Business

● ● ●

Whatever the mind of man can conceive and believe, it can achieve.

—NAPOLEON HILL, *THINK AND GROW RICH*

To be good is not enough when you dream of being great.

—NY SCHOOL OF ARTS POSTER

QUALITY SELLS. THE CUSTOMER OF the twenty-first century is very discerning. In addition, the business arena of the twenty-first century is tough and highly competitive. The main reason behind the recent popularity of healthcare tourism to Europe, America, and India is the search for quality. This point is key, so set up your healthcare business to deliver quality. The quality of your service is what will set you apart from the competition. You cannot afford to conduct your business with a carefree attitude. Never forget that a satisfied client is your best business strategy. In general, if people are paying for a service, they demand high quality. When you deliver on your promise of quality every time, trust develops. With trust comes a solid, good reputation, and your business becomes well known.

What constitutes a quality service or product? A quality health service or healthcare product is one that is effective in meeting the needs of the client. Quality services will be effective, safe, patient centered, timely, efficient, and respectful of dignity and individuality.

How Can Quality Be Measured?

The quality of the healthcare that is delivered can be measured from the following different perspectives:

- Interpersonal relationships
- Performance of the service
- Outcome of the service

For example, in an optician's practice, a *quality interpersonal relationship* would mean that the client is treated with courtesy and respect throughout an appointment or procedure. *Quality performance of service* would mean that the client is skillfully examined in a suitable facility and provided with appropriate information and guidance to make an informed choice about the solutions available. *Quality outcome* would mean that the chosen treatment option produces an effective solution to the problem. For example, if the patient has an eye defect and wearing the prescribed lenses adequately corrects his or her vision, that is a quality outcome.

There will be different parameters for different healthcare types. In general, there should be well-documented parameters that all the personnel in your organization are aware of and fully support. The parameters should include the following:

- Key performance indicators (KPIs)
- Client-satisfaction survey
- Complaint-handling procedure
- Regular audits to see that KPIs are met and, if not, mechanisms to correct the lapses

Seek Accreditation with Appropriate Bodies

Although accreditation is not mandatory for healthcare facilities in Nigeria, you should take the initiative to submit your business to an accreditation body relevant to your specialty.

CHAPTER 7

Managing and Growing the Healthcare Business

• • •

Be not afraid of growing slowly; be afraid only of standing still.

—CHINESE PROVERB

You will either step forward into growth,
or you will step back into safety.

—ABRAHAM MASLOW

To grow a business you need to spend time working on
and not simply working in the business, planning for the
future and taking an overview on what is going on.

—RICHARD BRANSON

ONCE YOUR ORGANIZATION IS UP and running, you must begin to work toward your business goals as stated in your business plan. There should be no room for complacency.

MANAGING YOUR BUSINESS
With regards to day-to-day management of the business, the following should be in place:

- A clinic diary where all appointments are recorded
- Regular open days and hours of business
- If it is a medical facility that runs a 24/7 service, clear work stops and out-of-hours (on-call) time starts
- Regular team meetings with set agendas (e.g., monthly meetings)

Promoting Your Business

Once you have opened your healthcare business, you should congratulate yourself. However, don't dwell too long in the self-congratulatory mode. Keep a watchful eye on how things are going. The systems that you have put in place and the efforts of your staff should put you on a sound footing, but you must not rest on your oars.

You should have a plan to promote your business. Don't be content with serving only your local community. You have spent time, effort, and money to set up a business delivering a quality service that will be useful to other clients far and wide. It is no time to be shy. You should develop a strategy to promote your business. Your strategies should include the following:

1. Investing in a good website to project you to the world—yes, to the world. That is the power of the Internet. It is powerful marketing tool.
2. Networking with other professionals locally and nationally
3. Utilizing social media such as Facebook and Twitter to connect with your clients and to promote your business to new clients
4. Advertising in newspapers, professional journals, popular blogs, on TV, and on websites of appropriate organizations and businesses

Building Your Team

A good team is essential for achieving your business goals. While you may be the prime entrepreneurial force of your organization, it will be helpful to find another colleague or two to team up with you. This is important for several reasons:

- It provides you with much-needed support in your business activities. The entrepreneurial pathway can be lonely.
- It is well known that two heads are better than one; this is so there can be synergy of ideas and efforts.
- Consider this scriptural endorsement for teamwork: "Two are better than one; because they have a good reward for their labor. For if they fall, the one will lift up his fellow; but woe to him that is alone when he falleth; for he hath not another to help him up. And if one prevail against him, two shall withstand him; and a threefold cord is not quickly broken" (Ecclesiastes 4:9–12).

GROWING YOUR BUSINESS

Don't let your business remain static. Ultimately, stasis will turn to decline. This is why you should plan actively for growth and expansion. Growth can be achieved in different ways:

- Through promotional activities whereby more people become aware of and use your services
- By introducing new services
- Through expanding your geographical reach by setting up a new branch either within your present town or city or outside of it. This is a major commitment and should receive thorough consideration before you come to a decision.

NETWORKING

Networking is the process by which business people and entrepreneurs meet to form business relationships and to recognize, create, or act upon business opportunities, to share information, and to seek potential partners for ventures. The avenues for networking are many and varied.

Traditional or face-to-face methods of networking include the following:

- Attending conferences and meetings of professionals
- Joining associations and interacting with the so-called old boys' network
- Participating in social events, church activities, and local community centers
- Contacting people and organizations through letters, e-mails, and phone calls

Social media has opened up countless possibilities for networking. Facebook, Twitter, and LinkedIn have all enhanced the ease of networking. Skype enables real-time meetings of participants across several continents.

Effective networking makes your product or service widely known, and personal contacts and interaction can facilitate the development of trust. However, networking for business growth should not be random or uncoordinated. It has to be strategic and focused. Networking activities have to be proactive, methodical, and persistent.

Networking will open doors to new people, but it is the cultivation of relationships that will bring a regular supply of new business. The good old courtesies (politeness, respect, keeping in touch through social activities) have not gone out of fashion. Together with trust and integrity, they form the fuel for long-lasting business relationships.

CHAPTER 8

Lessons from St. Jude's Entrepreneurial Journey

● ● ●

Never give in. Never give in. Never give in.

—Winston Churchill

Good ideas and Innovations must be driven
into existence by courageous patience.

—Admiral Rickover

A boat is safe in the harbor. But that is not what boats are for.

—Anonymous

I AM OFTEN ASKED WHAT has been my biggest satisfaction in my entrepreneurial journey. Many people expect me to say it is the financial reward, but that is not true. Of course, the money is good, very good, but it is not what has given me the most fulfillment.

My biggest satisfaction has been the opportunity to express my clinical skills and creativity unhindered by the political and corporate red tape inherent in the NHS.

My next best satisfaction is the opportunity to impact patients' lives positively by helping them procreate and have families of their own. This, I believe, is a basic human desire. In December 2012, we celebrated the birth of the thousandth baby born through treatment provided by St. Jude's Women's Hospital. The satisfaction I got from this landmark achievement goes beyond having money.

I have also derived immense pleasure from providing employment for many young and not-so-young men and women over the past fifteen years. I have also learnt some life lessons from some of these people.

I am also pleased that we have contributed to our local community in a purposeful way. We have made monetary donations to the local council and provided training opportunities for medical students, doctors, nurses, and midwives.

LESSONS LEARNT ALONG THE WAY

I started St. Jude's armed only with clinical skills and experience but little knowledge of business processes. As the business progressed, I had to resign from a well-paid NHS consultant post to focus on the clinic. Needless to say, this was very daunting. To make progress with the clinic, I had to teach myself different business subjects such as advertising and marketing, employment law and procedures, bookkeeping, basic accounting, and purchasing. The ideal would have been to employ different professionals to take care of the business side, but this was unaffordable at the early stage. All we could afford at the start was a secretary, who did most of the administrative duties. My young children provided additional receptionist and administrative duties on weekends when they were not in school. Fortunately, they had computer skills well beyond their ages. My son designed and managed the clinic's website, which served us for more than ten years! My son and two daughters produced our first set of patient-information leaflets using a desktop publisher. My wife, who is a university lecturer, also helped out with cleaning and housekeeping.

St. Jude's started in a rented suite of three rooms in a building that also housed two other businesses. In about two and a half years, we were able to buy our own building, with eight rooms and a separate annex consisting of three more rooms, a kitchen on the ground floor, and a first floor with a good-sized room and an adjoining sitting and storage area.

Two years later, an opportunity arose to buy another healthcare business located about an hour's drive from us. We saw this as an opportunity to increase our footprint, and by God's grace, we were able to purchase the premises and business the following year.

We are currently setting up a Women's Clinic in Nigeria, a country of about 170 million people crying out for innovation and creativity in healthcare provision.

St. Jude Hospitals and Clinics have been progressive and now generate a substantial amount of money. The financial reward makes a compelling case for embarking on a healthcare entrepreneurial venture. I believe the would-be healthcare entrepreneur can learn a lot from some of the challenges we have encountered. I will outline the lessons that can be learnt from our experience.

Ensure good record keeping.

The importance of good record keeping cannot be overemphasized. It is normally well emphasized during professional training, and many healthcare professionals do well in making notes of their interaction with clients. Often this requirement for good record keeping is not applied to other areas of their business. Good and accurate records must be kept in relation to income and expenditure, stock levels, client attendance, receipts of purchases, and invoices issued to clients. Financial records are essential for producing accurate accounts, which are mandatory for tax purposes. In the first few years of St. Jude's Clinic, bookkeeping records were not always complete. As a result, we often had to pay more tax than necessary.

Staff records are also essential for good personnel relations.

Seek advice early.

Being a good doctor or pharmacist or dentist is one thing; running a business is a different matter. Running a business involves many more skills that the healthcare professional is usually not equipped with. These are not taught as part of the professional training. It is therefore often necessary to seek advice from business consultants, accountants, and lawyers, to name a few sources of useful information. It is particularly important to seek legal advice when drawing up employment contracts for your employees and when drawing up agreements with business partners.

Don't overstretch yourself financially.

Starting a new venture will stretch your finances to a degree, but *don't be reckless*. Make sure you don't run out of cash; it will kill your business. This is where good business planning will help. You don't have to have all equipment in place from day one although obviously, you should have the essential equipment and materials to function safely and effectively. It may be possible to lease some of your equipment initially. With leasing, you are not tying down substantial capital, and you may even be able to pay the lease payments from cash flow.

You must control costs of staffing for your business. Only employ the minimum number of staff you need to deliver a good and safe service.

Seek collaboration.

You will achieve so much more through collaboration with colleagues or other similar businesses. It will definitely help to bring in a colleague for backup and support. It can be lonely as an entrepreneur. The colleague doesn't necessarily have to be offered shares in the business; you can offer payment on a pro rata basis. If both parties are happy, you can then offer part-ownership (shares), which can be any percentage that reflects his or her role and involvement.

Negotiate favorable terms with your suppliers.

It will help your cash flow to negotiate discounts on items you purchase and the duration of credit terms. Having agreed to terms of payment, you must make sure you keep to them. Late payments for the goods you have purchased will quickly erode trust and bring your credibility into question. Remember that your supplier also needs cash on a timely basis to run his or her business.

DEVELOP A GOOD RELATIONSHIP WITH YOUR BANK RELATIONSHIP MANAGER.

It certainly helps to have a good relationship with your bank through your relationship manager. Provide regular updates on the progress of the business. Your manager will already have some idea of how your business is doing from your bank statements. Invite your manager to come and see the business and meet your staff.

If you buy him or her lunch every now and again, your manager will look more favorably on your request if and when you ask for an increase in your overdraft or a loan. This is a basic act to nurture good relationships, both in business and personal relationships. I do not consider this gesture as bribery or corruption. It is common in the United Kingdom.

BE COMMITTED TO CONTINUOUS PROFESSIONAL DEVELOPMENT (CPD) FOR ALL STAFF.

The key to success in healthcare business is lifelong learning. Therefore, you must have a plan for continuous professional development. It will ensure that your skills are up to date.

BE DETERMINED TO OVERCOME THE SO-CALLED "NIGERIAN FACTOR."

It must be said that Nigeria is not the easiest place to do business. What has come to be termed the "Nigerian factor" is an unfortunate mixture of problems such as the unreliable power supply, the unreliable water supply, bribery and corruption, and counterfeit drugs.

You can't run a healthcare business (or any business for that matter) in Nigeria without having your own generator. In our setup, we use the generator most of the time, especially when we are carrying out procedures in theatre and absolutely must have an uninterrupted supply of power. Using your own generator incurs a high cost, of course, since diesel fuel is expensive.

Most businesses, and indeed most households, have their own boreholes to provide a reliable water supply. Again, this adds to the cost of doing business, a cost that is invariably passed on to clients.

Many agree that corruption is the main impediment to progress in many facets of Nigerian society. It is probably at the core of the chronic lack of all utilities (electricity, water, and so on) and poor healthcare facilities in Nigeria. It is a complex issue, and many hope that President Muhammadu Buhari will succeed in his war against corruption.

The problem of counterfeit drugs has particular relevance to healthcare businesses. NAFDAC (the National Agency for Food and Drug Administration and Control) has schemes to check that drugs are genuine. If in doubt, you must contact NAFDAC.

CONCLUSION: SUCCESS — YOUR DESTINATION

Winning starts with beginning

—ROBERT SCHULLER

Be daring. Be first. Be different.

—ANITA RODDICK, FOUNDER OF 'THE BODY SHOP'

The purpose of a job or career change should be
that of seeking greater self-fulfillment

—ANONYMOUS

Nothing more frustrating than being dependent on
someone else for the opportunity to succeed

—EDWIN LAND, FOUNDER OF POLAROID CORPORATION

HEALTHCARE ENTREPRENEURSHIP HAS A VITAL role to play in improving the provision and quality of healthcare services in Nigeria. The rewards of a successful private setup include career fulfillment and financial reward. The days of a two-room clinic in your father's house are long gone. New healthcare organizations should be based on a carefully considered plan and be professionally run with clearly defined objectives. There are advantages in involving one or more colleagues, as there is strength in numbers. Your operating systems should be based on international best practices. There should be ambition to grow and expand the business.

Some say success, like happiness, defies definition. This is because success has many facets. The simple dictionary definition of success is the achievement of something desired, planned, or attempted.

In your entrepreneurial endeavor, you can claim success for several things:

- Taking the bold move to step out of the boat and set up your own business
- Providing a service or product to help people
- Delivering a service in an innovative way, thereby making your contribution to healthcare quality improvement
- Earning a living from your own handiwork
- Providing employment to others and therefore making a contribution to the national economy

If you follow the counsel of this book, you will bask in your success for a long time to come. In the unlikely event that things don't work out, take heart; you are not a failure. Through your experiences, you have learnt lessons that will help to make your next venture a success.

In closing, I recommend that you digest these words of wisdom from Dr. Mike Murdock, the world-renowned preacher and president of the Wisdom Center in Texas, United States: "An uncommon life is decided by what you are willing to overcome. An uncommon life is not a life without mistakes. The Bible says all men fail. All have sinned and come short of the glory of God. A just man will fall down seven times but he will rise again (Proverbs 24:16). All men fall; the great ones get back up."

USEFUL BOOKS

Blank, Steve, and Bob Dorf. *The Startup Owner's Manual: The Step-by-Step Guide for Building a Great Company*. K&S Ranch Publishing Co., 2012.

Carnegie, Dale. *How to Win Friends and Influence People*. London: Vermilion, 2006.

Ciuci Consulting (Lore Muriana, Israel Tommy, and Chukwuka Monye). *Outbound Medical Tourism: Result of a Poor Healthcare System*. June 2012

Cohen, David, and Brad Feld. *Do More Faster: TechStars Lessons to Accelerate Your Startup*. Hoboken, NJ: John Wiley & Sons, 2011.

Craven, Robert. *Kick-Start Your Business: Virgin Business Guides*. London: Virgin Publishing, Ltd., 2001.

Hill, Napoleon. *The Law of Success—In Sixteen Lessons*. Radford, VA: Wilder Publications, 2011.

Hill, Napoleon. *Think and Grow Rich*. Radford, VA: Wilder Publications, 2007.

Hseih, Tony. *Delivering Happiness: A Path to Profits, Passion, and Purpose*. New York: Hachette Book Group, 2010.

Johnson, Steven. *Where Good Ideas Come From: The Seven Patterns of Innovation*. New York: Penguin Books, 2011.

Parks, Steve. *How to Be an Entrepreneur: The Six Secrets of Self-Made Success*. Harlow: Pearson Education Ltd., 2006.

Shell, G. Richard. *Success, Your Way: Do What You're Meant to Do.* New York: Penguin, 2013.

Webb, Philip, and Sandra Webb. *The Small Business Handbook: The Entrepreneur's Definitive Guide to Starting and Growing a Business.* Upper Saddle River, NJ: Prentice Hall, 2001.

USEFUL WEBSITES

www.bplans.co.uk

http://www.entrepreneurs.healthcare

https://hqijournal.wordpress.com

http://qualityhealthcareacademy.blogspot.com

www.paloalto.com/uk

www.ingramcontent.com/pod-product-compliance
Lightning Source LLC
Chambersburg PA
CBHW070412190526
45169CB00003B/1221